BeautifulRightNow.com
Presents:

The Beauty Secrets Doctors Save For Celebrities

Dr. Bonnie Marting DNP ARNP

DISCLAIMER

No graphics, photos, texts nor links to or from YearsErased.com or BeautifulRightNow.com, whether authored by Dr. Bonnie Marting DNP, ARNP, or another person (professional or otherwise), shall be construed as an attempt to offer or render a medical opinion or otherwise engage in the practice of medicine or transmitting of medical advice.

No warranty whatsoever is made by Years Erased, Inc. or Dr. Bonnie Marting DNP, ARNP, that any of the subjects covered in this book are accurate in every given situation. There is no assurance whatsoever that any statement contained (or cited) in this book regarding medical or other matters, is precise, up to date, or will not cause harm in certain specific situations.

Some statements in this book may address, comment on, or attempt to explain medical procedures or treatments. **These statements may or may not be accurate, based on your specific situation.** If accurate in some particular instance, they still may not apply to you or your symptoms/problems. **Consult your medical professional before going forward with anything contained in this book.**

ALL information contained within this book, medical and otherwise, is, at best, of a general nature and cannot substitute for the advice of a medical professional that has seen and personally advised you regarding your specific problem and/or symptom.

4300 US Hwy 1 203-262
Jupiter, FL 33477

www.BeautifulRightNow.com

This book of beauty secrets
is dedicated to you.

TABLE OF CONTENTS

FOREWORD

Like many people, I went through most of my life ignoring the importance of our skin. Anatomy classes taught me that skin was the body's largest organ, but I still didn't "connect the dots." I baked in the sun when I could, and thought having a great tan was really cool. I paid little attention to the warning signs. I guess I thought I was going to look young forever. Funny how the years, and a bit of wisdom, changes all that unrealistic thinking.

But finally the light flickered on. And this light wasn't from a sunlamp—it was from the courses I took in college. When I studied cosmetic skin care medicine, I realized how much our skin reflected choices we made years ago—yesterday, today and every day since.

My own skin began showing signs of neglect and abuse about the same time I started studying my specialty. Therefore, I pretty much became my own "test lab." The more I studied, the more my passion grew regarding proper skin care and rejuvenation.

With that in mind, I began mentally writing this book. It took some time to get it all on paper, but I knew it was something I had to complete. Very few publications I found had the "real truth." But if you wanted to find a bunch of advertising scams, lies, and untruths, they were everywhere. I thought to myself—how does the average person know what they can believe and what they should stay away from? With so much marketing hype on the market for skin creams and formulas, it was horribly frustrating for someone in my profession to see the blatant lies being manufactured and sold to the average consumer. As my passion for skin health grew and saw years erased from my own appearance, I realized I was truly onto something remarkable.

My goal had become a reality! Without plastic surgery, I had taken years off my appearance and created younger, healthier, more beautiful skin in the process. I looked younger and felt great. This book is the culmination of that research and experience. My techniques have been tested on thousands of patients in my office, and of course, on myself.

I was blessed to study under some of the finest practitioners and learn firsthand what works, what doesn't, and how to properly combine procedures and treatments based on individual needs.

For years now, I have had my own practice and every day I see patients just like you leave my office feeling great and looking younger. Some say they feel like they've entered a time machine and literally turned back the clock. Many love to look at themselves in the mirror now, whereas before they dreaded the reflection that greeted them every morning. It's unbelievable how a part of their youthful enthusiasm has been returned.

Your face, your skin, and your overall appearance is like a window to the world. When people see you, they must look through the glass to see what you are really like. Don't have foggy, smudged, dirty panels or broken panes. Feel and look fabulous inside and out. Everyone wants to be Beautiful Right Now. Look as young as you feel. I'll show you how. That's what makes it all worthwhile!

This book, *Beauty Secrets Doctors Save For Celebrities,* is the first in a series of short books to help you better understand your skin. Making your skin healthier and look younger is something I'm passionate about. I hope this book will guide you on your quest to becoming Beautiful Right Now.

Please do not hesitate to give me your thoughts and share your story. You are important to me. It's why this book was written.

Sincerely,

Dr. Bonnie Marting DNP ARNP

PART ONE

Mirror, Mirror On The Wall...

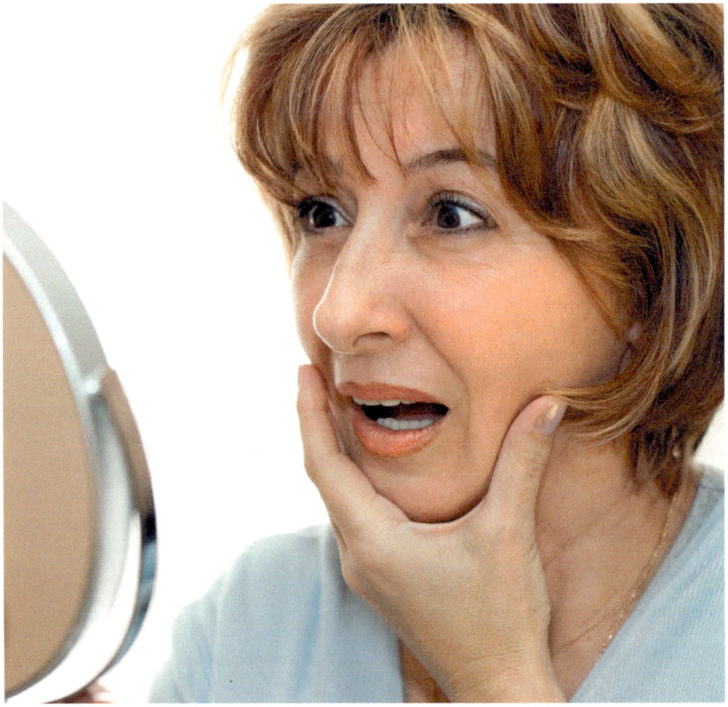

This Looks Bad, Who Can I Call?

If beauty is only skin deep, why do we work so hard to make it look better? Because...it's the first thing you see when you look in the mirror; it's the first thing that people see when they meet you; and it certainly affects the way you feel about yourself.

I read an interesting statement: "Every person over the age of 40 has a voice inside them saying 'What happened to me?' "

I believe it. It seems like just yesterday that our skin was smooth and tight. Now it's beginning to take on a look we don't really want to name—but we know what it's called. We look tired and worn out; we're less vibrant and youthful. The glow is gone and has been replaced by sagging, lines and wrinkles. Gasp—could it be? Are we actually getting old? Let me reassure you of your sanity. It's not in your head. Something really is happening to your skin. It didn't happen overnight, but can seem like it if you've been ignoring the signs and the mirror.

When we are young, skin elasticity and tightness are controlled by plentiful amounts of tightly wound collagen fibers. These provide an abundant nutrient supply through healthy blood vessels, and are coupled with a rich layer of subcutaneous (under the skin) fatty tissue. It's that perfect weaving that provides a smooth, soft look. Picture a plump, glowing toddler and you'll have a picture of perfect skin in your head.

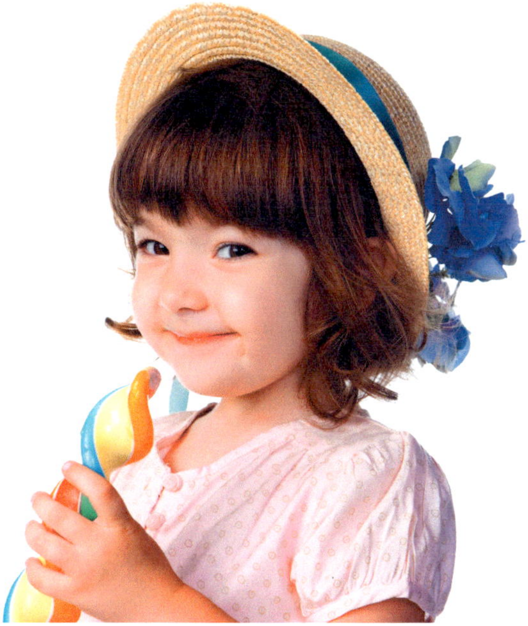

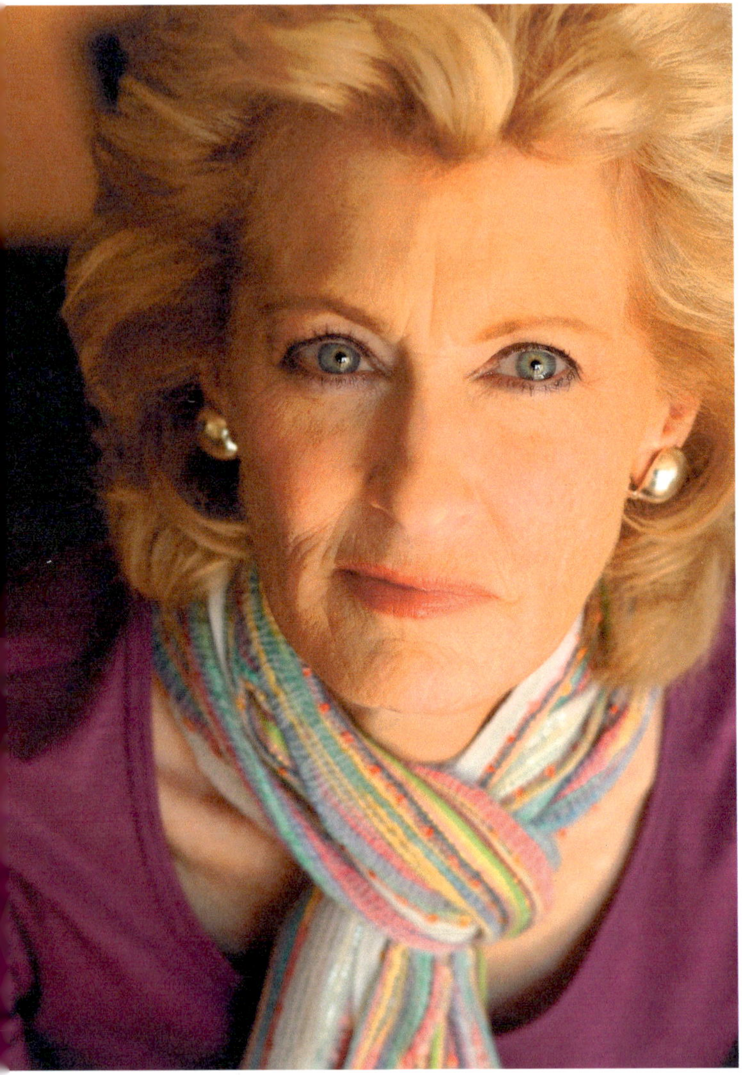

As we age, collagen, subcutaneous tissue, blood vessels, and elastic fibers begin to disappear. The skin becomes thinner, more fragile, and non-elastic. We may also see dark spots, and some areas become almost coarse to the touch. What we see is our skin beginning to "age."

These signs can come as early as age 30. As collagen loss increases, those slight, crepe-like lines remain, and not just when you're tired. At the same time, a mild loss of facial fat may make the face more angular, especially at the cheek bones. Later on, a narrowing of the face becomes apparent as collagen, fat (and even bone) are lost to time and degradation. Menopause and loss of estrogen increase the damage, as the rate of fat loss escalates and sagginess becomes more apparent. Prior sun history makes our skin deteriorate even more rapidly.

Yes, this is bad news, but better news is ahead. While this progression cannot be entirely stopped, we are seeing almost miraculous results from new technologies and procedures that can make it appear as if you had Years Erased.

I'll show you how to look like the "After" pictures—not the "Before." You can literally take ten, twenty, or even more years off your appearance—without having a facelift!

But first, what are you trying to correct? Did you do something to get to this place or were you genetically predisposed to age before your time?

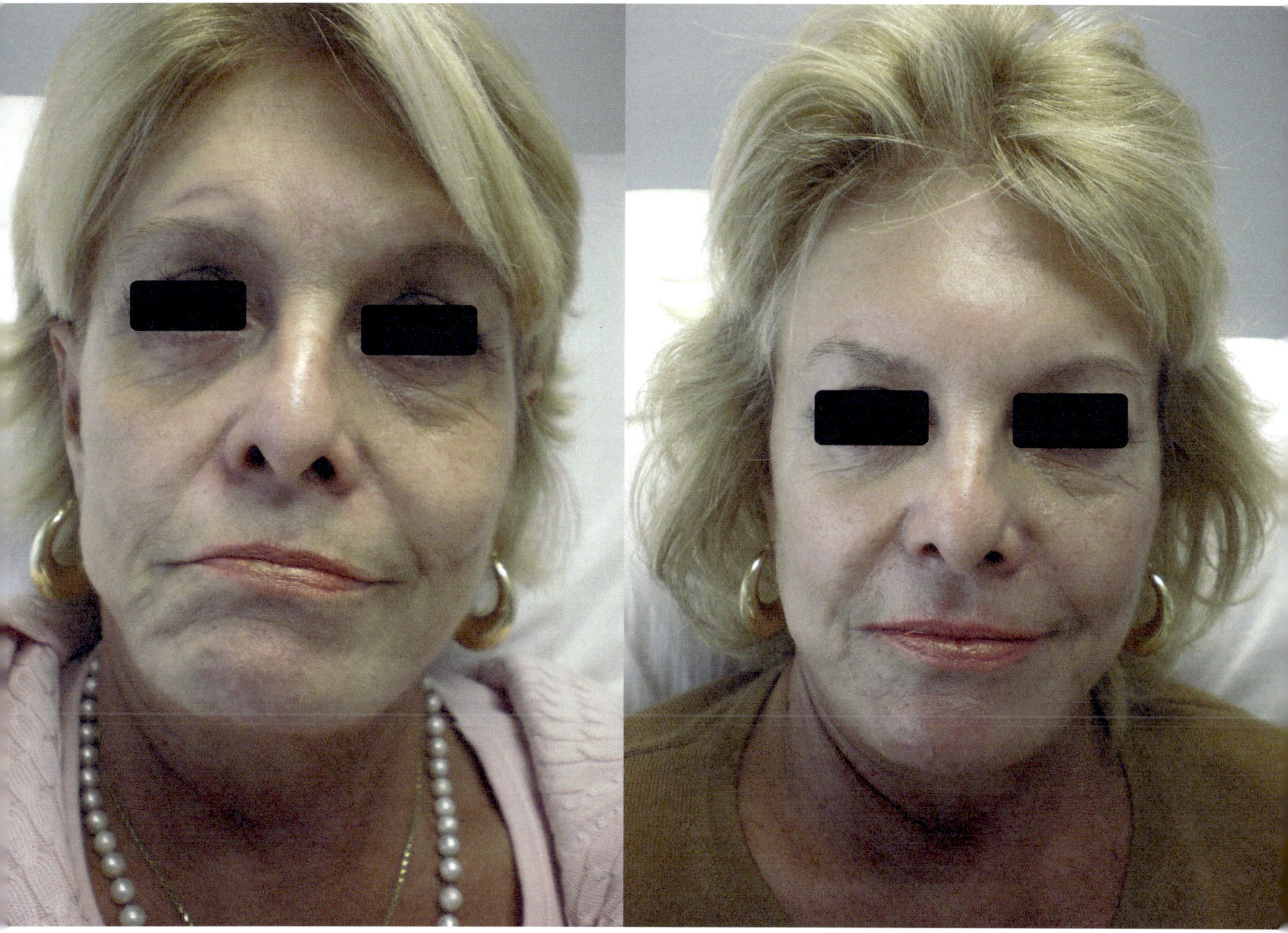

Before After

Has Your Past Caught Up With You?

Unfortunately, as we go through life, constant micro-offenses occur to your skin. This is a fancy way of saying all those little things we've done or ignored in our past have been building up and now we're paying for them. Think of how many times we don't wear a visor or hat, or how often we go outside without sunscreen. Maybe you popped a pimple or two in your youth, or frequently go to bed with makeup and not wash your face. These are just a few of the little micro-offenses I'm talking about.

We know now that sun exposure received at a young age is far more harmful than previously realized. Ultraviolet rays from the sun, specifically UVA and UVB, cause a harmful amount of free-radical formation to our skin with <u>every</u> exposure.

Free Radicals

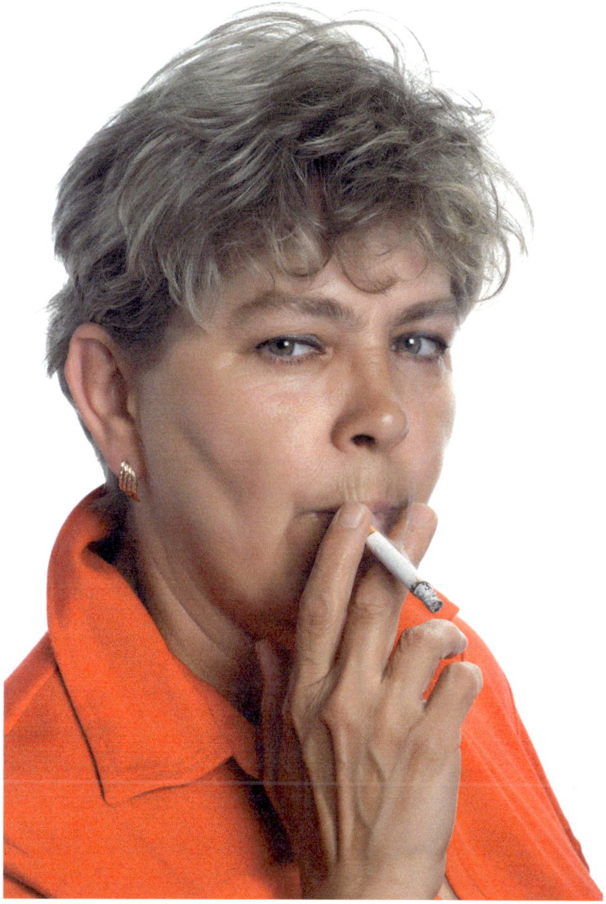

The term "free radicals" is thrown around like a marketing mantra today. So many products, labeled as antioxidants, say they eliminate free radicals, but what do free radicals actually do, and why are they so bad?

Simply put, free radicals are organic molecules responsible for aging, tissue damage, and possibly some diseases. These free radical molecules are very unstable. They need an oxygen atom to survive. As they desperately seek this oxygen atom, they damage surrounding cells in their wild, vicious search. At the same time, they rob other molecules of the beloved oxygen they too are depending on. This causes extensive damage over time and accelerates what we call the "aging process."

What creates free radicals?

Take a guess...

Free radicals are generated by:

- **Smoking**
- **Environmental factors**
  - Excessive sun: UV rays from the sun and tanning beds
  - Pollution: factories burning fossil fuels, pesticides, mining operations, combustion engine exhaust, etc.
- **Natural metabolism**
  (Just living can create free radicals)

Skin Survivors Don't Get Voted Off The Island. They Stick Around!

Our skin is really smart, as are most of our organs. Twenty four hours a day, seven days a week, our bodies work toward self-preservation. Skin, like other organs, has protection built in, but unfortunately it can ultimately be depleted if we don't take action to help the struggle.

As skin attempts to protect itself, the damage is still occurring and eventually becomes visible. One of skin's most obvious warning signals is sunburn pain. Regardless of whether the burn turns into a tan—it is still a sunburn and bad for you. This initial burn tells you something is being harmed. Your body creates discomfort that is hopefully an incentive to either avoid the sun or at least utilize sunscreen protection.

Unfortunately this warning is not always listened to, resulting in skin that becomes permanently damaged—both visually and on the cellular level. Eventually the stratum corneum, which is the very top layer of dead keratin cells, will become thicker. This is because it's the skin's only defense. By becoming denser, it becomes more impenetrable in an attempt to prevent further damage to the delicate tissue below. Eventually this continued bombarding overcomes the stratum corneum's efforts to protect the tissue below and damage occurs in varying degrees. This is what we interpret as "aging skin." You can see some pretty bad examples of this process in the Sunbelt areas of our country, especially Florida and the Southwest.

PART TWO

Let's Talk Ancestry

Do You Have Lighter Skinned Ancestors In Your Family Tree?

Believe it or not, ancestral heritage is a question I always ask a new patient. It's important to know your background to determine the best protection and treatment. Each of us holds genetic clues that provide information as to why our skin and appearance has responded like it has. Our skin will react differently to certain procedures versus someone with a different DNA. In other words, we're not all alike just because we're humans.

Some individuals are "ancestrally" lucky. A certain amount of built-in protection comes with their heritage. We know that while African-Americans can burn, they have much more protection than the average Caucasian. Greeks, many Italians, some Asians, and Native Americans also possess these skin-protection characteristics. Their darker skin color usually means they will have some hereditary advantages built into their family tree. Other people are not so lucky; those with Northern European ancestry are most susceptible to sun damage.

"Some individuals are 'ancestrally' lucky. They have a certain amount of built in protection with their heritage."

One interesting medical fact that supports the heritage issue is the rate of skin cancer in Australia. The highest in the world! The reason is deceptively simple. Most of the original migration to Australia came from Northern Europe. Coming from an area with very little sun compared to Australia, these people were thrust into this sun-drenched continent and even today are paying the price of having no built-in "ancestral" protection.

What would the average Australian look like if she had been protected from the sun? Nicole Kidman comes to mind. She has beautiful skin, and obviously has been protected since childhood from harmful sun rays.

PART THREE

What You Can Do On Your Own

There is a lot you can do for yourself. First, let's start changing the progression of what's happening today in your skin. If we don't do that initially, things will continue to get worse.

There are many things under our control that can stop and even reverse what has been happening to your skin. Some are as simple as keeping a daily skin regimen (kind of like gym for your skin). Actually, the "mainstays" of skin fitness are the same as you would see in a general fitness program.

Stop Smoking

I know it is easy for me to say, but you must make a serious effort to stop smoking if you truly want healthy skin. Toxins produced by smoking greatly decrease the body's ability to nourish cells. It may interest you to know that many plastic surgeons feel so strongly about the unhealthy factors related to smoking that they will not consider operating on a smoker. Everything from the actual surgery to overall outcome (including healing time) is negatively affected by smoking.

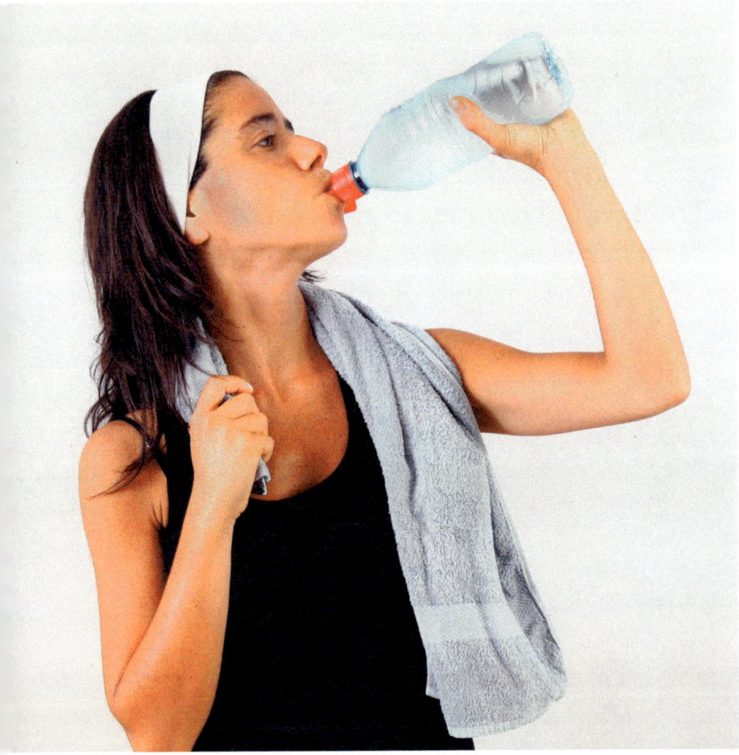

Drink Water

Abundant hydration is necessary. While it's possible to overdose on water, it's also highly unlikely. Most of us truly do not get enough water. We get plenty of soft drinks and coffee, but not pure water. And, it need not be bottled. Tap water is fine.

While it is generally understood that a body doesn't transfer water directly to the skin as we drink, our bodies still use hydration in many ways, skin health and replication being one.

Exercise

Aerobic exercise is great. It increases circulation to all of your organs including your skin. By the way, it came as a real surprise to me in medical school when I found out that skin is our largest organ—both in size and weight! I don't know what I thought it was, but I did not associate my skin as an organ. (Thankfully I wasn't the only one who didn't know that answer, as most people named their heart, kidneys, or brain when asked what their largest organ was). Anyway, back to our skin.

Aerobic exercise increases oxygen, and oxygenation is one of your body's great nutrients. It also encourages a sense of well-being. (That's why oxygen bars are popping up all over). Good exercise can lead directly to better, healthier skin by increasing oxygen flow.

Diet

I think we all know that a diet rich in vegetables, fruits, and proteins will make us healthier and feel better. Often we (me included) do not pay careful enough attention to what goes in our mouths. But we should monitor this diligently because it is important.

Our country has a diet way too heavy in fats and carbohydrates. I have nothing against carbs, but they need to be balanced. Metabolic syndrome, a combination of medical disorders that increase the risk of developing cardiovascular disease and diabetes, is out of control. The number of overweight people and obese individuals in our population is skyrocketing. (Note: There is a difference between just being overweight, and being considered obese. It is based on your BMI—body mass index. No one should aspire to be a weight that is unhealthy—no matter what rating you get on a chart—so take note of where you are on the scales and on the index.)

A diet high in fat and carbs doesn't contain the necessary antioxidants your body desires. That type of diet can't squelch the thirst for the oxygen atom. This results in an imbalance of free radicals as discussed earlier. The maladies from being overweight create lots of free radicals searching for their oxygen atom. As we learned earlier, this free radical imbalance can be harmful to your skin.

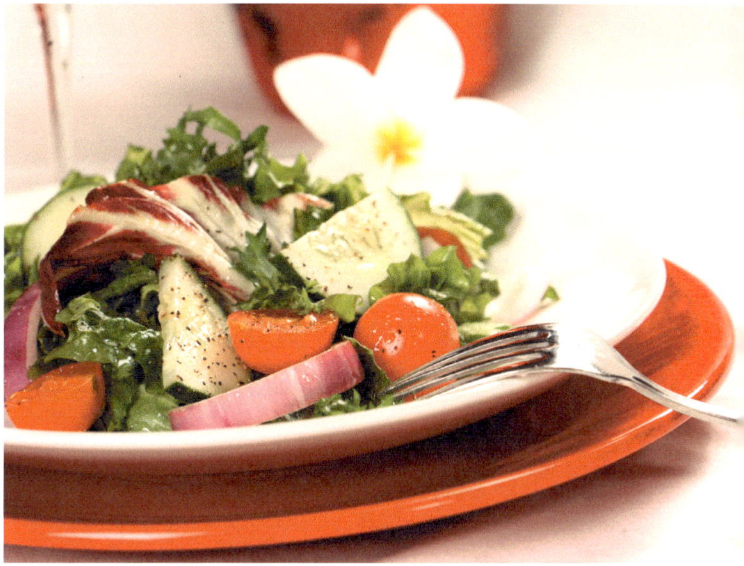

What Can You Do Now?

Think of your body and skin as one. Consciously drink water and choose your foods wisely. Get some aerobic exercise. Yoga is phenomenal, but should not be substituted for aerobic exercise.

PART FOUR

What Does "Evidence Based" Really Mean?

When I see a new patient, we usually go over what changes they would like to see. Then, we talk about what they are currently doing for skin care. Many will share their experiences with "quick fix" topically applied (smear on your skin) products. While there are a lot of good products that will help change your skin, the vast majority will change nothing except money from your bank account to theirs.

Let's listen in on a typical new patient consult:

Me: *"Hi, I'm Bonnie Marting, it's a pleasure to meet you. What brings you in today?"*

Patient: "Well, I wanted to see if there was something that would get rid of these lines on my face and maybe make my skin a little tighter."

Me: *"Well, there are a lot of things we could do, depending on what areas you want to work on. What are you doing now?"*

Patient: "Oh, I am using ________ (fill in the blank). I used to use _______ (fill in the blank) but this new formula came out, so I thought I would give it a try. I have been using it for a while and it seemed to work at first, but now I am not seeing anything at all. It just seemed to stop working, but I really noticed a difference at first. The lady behind the counter really recommended it highly. She said it had this process that used several products at the same time to get rid of these bad places and an anti-oxidant to bring back tone in my skin."

Me: *"I am not sure I have heard of that product. What differences could you see when you first used it?"*

{Sometimes they name a product, a website, or some other obscure name that, quite honestly, I have never heard of. I am always amazed at the amount of new things on the market, most of which are simply old ointments with a new name and label.}

Patient: "Well, my skin seemed to even out a little bit and I think some of the lines maybe went away, but I really wonder if it was worth the $128 I paid. And it was on sale! These lines are back and now I'm getting these (pointing to the side of her face where she has crepe-like, basket-weave indentations) lines that make me look awful. Is there anything we can do about them?"

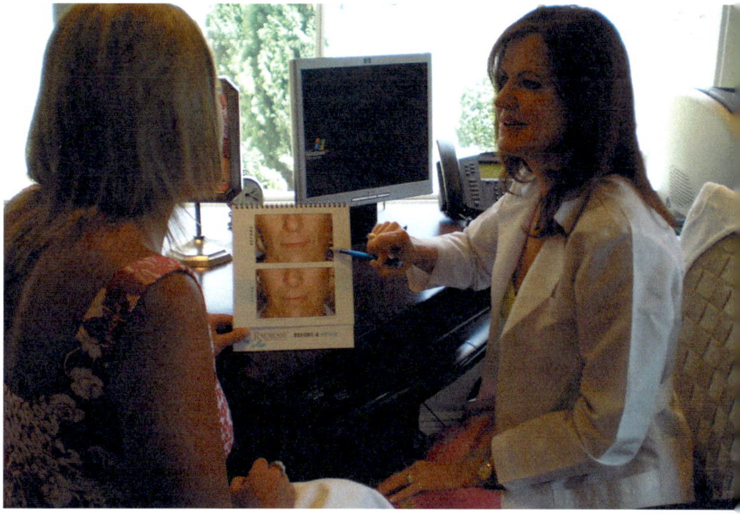

The answer to this question is almost always yes. There is something we can do, but first we will need to treat the problem instead of just the symptom showing up on the skin.

Don't take that the wrong way! I am not condemning my patients for trying all those products. I have seen some of the ads, and many are highly convincing. But unfortunately, almost all are highly priced, with little or no real evidence to back up their claims.

Now let's talk about Evidence Based.

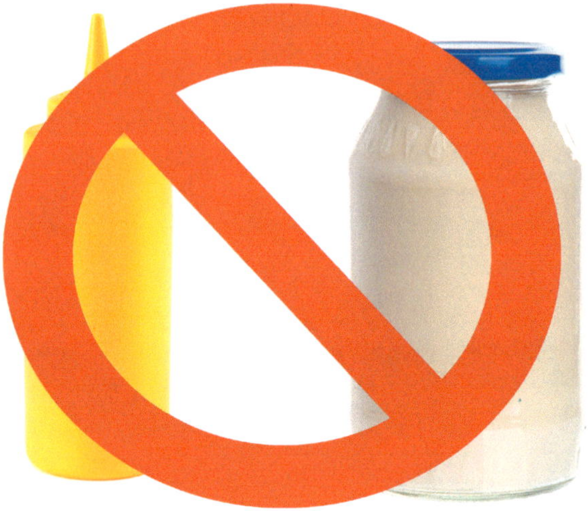

Evidenced-Based Products Or Procedures

Everyone has their "pet peeves," and I admit non-evidence based solutions is one of my biggest! I get so irritated when I read these claims and know they are not based on any shred of real evidence.

A real study is conducted by a medically correct independent source using a blind study where no participant is aware of what the product is or the desired outcome. The test is audited and results are documented thoroughly over a large user population. This will produce results that are factual and not skewed.

Some of the ads I see make me feel like I am supposed to buy a product based on its smoothness or depth of shine or some other criteria that has nothing to do with healthy skin. It's your skin we are dealing with, not furniture polish! Never buy a product based on "how smooth your skin feels," or the "tingle." Mayonnaise can make skin smooth, and mustard can add the tingle!

By the way, before and after photos don't count as evidence-based documentation. Computer editing or lighting can work wonders. Everyone knows what Adobe® Photoshop® is capable of nowadays. And what's with all the before pictures of the women with washed-out hair and no makeup being compared to the after photo where they have a completely new hairstyle and full makeup on? Of course they're going to look better. I mean seriously, are these meant to persuade us?

To compound the problem of getting really good products over the counter, many of the busiest cosmetic counters are more about commissioned sales than offering quality evidence-based skin care. Did you think that nice lady behind the counter really pushed that product on you because it works so great, or because she had a car payment due this month? Commission sales pitches are not the best way to judge whether or not a product will work for you.

"Clinically and medically evidence-based studies should be demanded for every skin product or procedure."

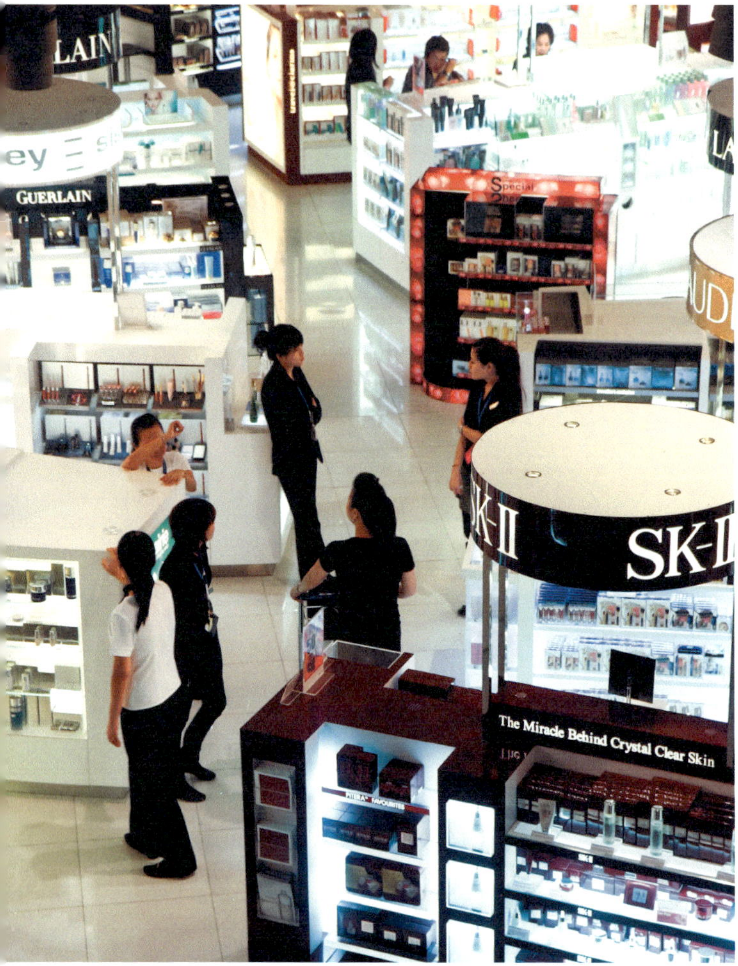

Evidence Based Solutions

Quality skin care products containing the proper ingredient dosage for your skin needs can only be found in your practitioner's office. Over-the-counter skin care products usually have low amounts of all the key ingredients, but that's just so they can claim them. There is rarely enough of the key ingredients contained within to actually complete the desired outcome. This is because their formulation has to fit anyone that buys their product. Based on that fact alone, if you find something that starts to work, it may take forever to see real long lasting results. If you try to "double up" on the amount you use, you may be risking skin damage.

Another risk of over-the-counter products is in finding good quality assistance. If you do see some change (positive or negative) and need advice on what to do next, your salesperson will have no medical background to help you get to the next level of skin health or diagnose your problem. So, as the marketing department wanted in the beginning, you just keep buying the same product over and over until you are introduced to the next "latest and greatest."

This is another reason why a professional in the field of cosmetic skin rejuvenation and skin care can be such a great find to you, not only financially but also emotionally. Your medical skin care practitioner is trained and educated to know what's happening inside your skin, and may be able to speed up the rejuvenation process for you by prescribing a more potent product. They might also prescribe a particular ingredient in combination with another. Professional care, coupled with proper follow up and evidence-based treatment is necessary for healthy, younger looking skin.

"The field of cosmetic skin rejuvenation and skin care can be a great find, not only financially but also emotionally."

PART FIVE

To Cream Or Not To Cream, That Is The Question

I see many of the same symptoms every day. Dry skin, redness, crepe-like marking (especially when you "gather" the skin), fine lines, wrinkles and dark spots.

When any of these symptoms are visible, your skin needs something that will achieve correction, not just an attempt to "moisturize" the skin to the point of saturation.

As we discussed earlier, your stratum corneum (exposed top layer of skin) has been attempting to protect the underlying skin structure by becoming denser, less elastic, and more waterproof. It does this by calling on the keratin cells inside the stratum corneum to make a barrier. As keratin cells become hard and less elastic, your skin will begin to appear mottled with any or all the symptoms mentioned earlier.

What's actually happening when these signs occur is your skin crying for help. Regular "moisturizing" creams or potions simply cannot penetrate this abused top layer to answer that cry. The most you can hope for is a slight "bloating" of this layer, which may appear to faintly decrease the visible lines for a short amount of time. This course of action will never get you to the goal you're looking for—long-term results that will have you erasing years off your appearance and looking more Beautiful Right Now. Relying on moisturizers simply wastes valuable time and money. Your efforts would be much better spent receiving proper treatment from a professional. And honestly, you should get started right away—the sooner you start, the better.

Getting Through the Stratum Corneum

As you can see by the diagram, the skin has three Skin Layers: Epidermis, Dermis, and Subcutaneous Fat Tissue.

The stratum corneum is the exposed layer in the epidermis (top layer) of your skin. It's very thin and has a tough job trying to protect everything below its surface. Being totally exposed to

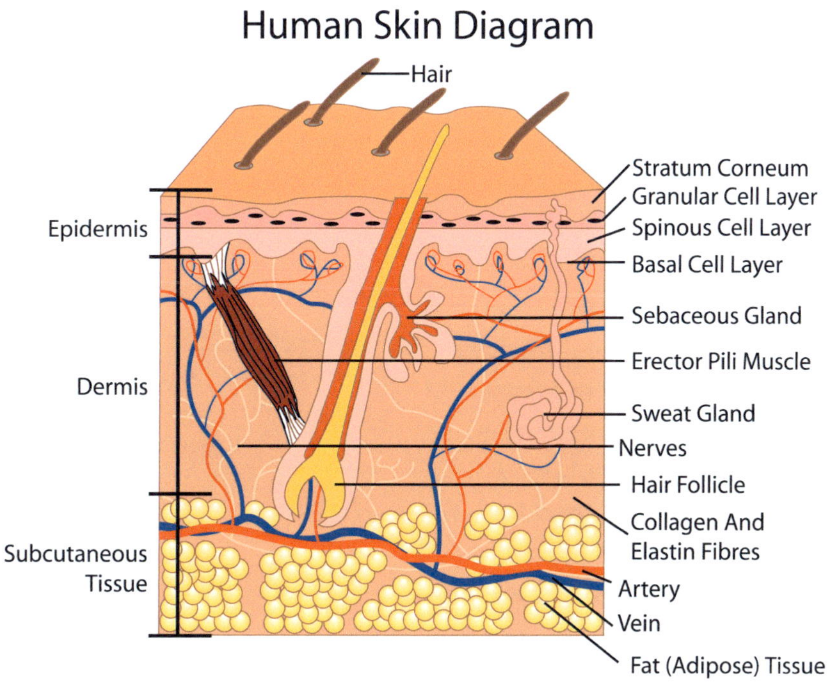

sun and free-radical damage, it becomes thicker in texture and more mottled in appearance as keratin cells become hard and less elastic. The resulting dark spots and thickness of these cells are its only defense. In reality, it's just trying to protect you as it is bombarded by sun and other free-radical damage.

So, What Do I Need?

Many patients come in asking for treatments they have heard about to improve their skin. That's a great starting point, and leads me to the part of my practice I truly love. I'm not one of those doctors who want to give you a quick prescription or pill. I don't do the traditional slice and dice of some practitioners. I like to get to know my patients. I want to understand what is important to them and why they are sitting in front of me. By taking my time and asking relevant questions, I am able to go over all the alternatives available. Some are topical, some involve laser resurfacing, and many involve injectables. Never will you read here that I recommend a surgical face lift or radical surgery to make you look younger. It is simply not necessary when there are so many other great products and procedures on the market now. And the best part is—if done properly by a trained professional, you can achieve the look you desire and erase years off your appearance and improve your overall skin health in the process.

So what do I recommend first? In many cases, I suggest methods to alter the current cell replication. By doing this change, you can see satisfying results quickly.

PART SIX

Glycolics, Retinoids, and Antioxidants (All the Good Stuff)

You and your practitioner will work together to help your skin recover and look younger. Not by using a temporary Band-Aid, but by using evidence-based solutions that start decreasing the resistance of the keratin in the stratum corneum. I know it sounds counter-productive to reduce resistance, but this is a necessary first step. Also, you need to stay sun free as we work together to allow other aspects of the treatment to do their job on the layers below where the healing occurs.

Our goal is to speed replication of good cells, which can retard the growth of mutations (pre-cancers and skin cancers) caused by previous violations of free radicals in your skin. All this may sound foreign to you now, but we will talk more about it as we go on.

Glycolics, The Boring Alternative

Unfortunately, glycolics are boring. They don't have a chic, trendy name. They have, however, been studied for years, and are truly a mainstay of the beauty industry. Their one drawback is when first applied, they can be a bit unnerving as your skin may appear like it has a mild to moderate sunburn. This happens because glycolic is the smallest molecule of the alpha-hydroxy family, and penetrates better than most. This rejuvenation is what makes your skin react as if you have sunburn.

"In the hands of a competent practitioner, I have seen glycolics literally take years of damage away."

After the redness disappears, your dermal depth will increase and the "structure" of the skin, where your collagen is, will regain some of its youthful elasticity.

This rather complicated reaction, and the fact that you want a competent practitioner to be your guide through the process, is why you will not find the good stuff over the counter.

Unfortunately, what I prescribe isn't in a fancy package. Prescription glycolics work, but don't expect pretty boxes and fancy bottles. They're not meant to look good on your vanity, but they do perform miracles on your skin. They deliver results that science and clinical trials have proven effective.

Glycolic, in an amount carefully prescribed for you, has been tested in the delivery vehicle (the main substance that contains the solution) for many years and proven itself to be a great skin rejuvenator. Many over-the-counter products have a small amount of this key ingredient. Unfortunately, it is almost always diluted by a fragrance or oil-based delivery vehicle that would take gallons of the stuff, and a full year to make any difference. So, forget the fancy packaging and get the results you're looking for from a trained practitioner and not a makeup counter saleslady.

The Retinoid Miracle

Retinoids are probably the greatest drugs ever created for skin rejuvenation. They have the ability to turn cells over even faster than glycolics, which as we just found out, will increase your dermal depth. Retinoids will also increase vascular activity which is pure nourishment to your skin, reducing fine lines and wrinkles.

Both glycolics and retinoids are effective, but retinoids are *drugs* and should be taken with care, as should any drug. They can only be prescribed by a licensed health care provider with prescriptive authority. Also, like any drug, retinoids have some side effects.

First, they may seem harsh and give your skin some mild discomfort. This may last for a few weeks but will decrease as time goes by. If by chance you become pregnant, a retinoid should immediately be discontinued. If you are trying to get pregnant, do not start with a retinoid. It would be best to stick to a glycolic-based product during this time. A few examples of retinoid brand names include, but are not limited to:

- Retin-A®
- Retin-A Micro®
- Tazorac®
- Avage®
- Differin®

"As a side benefit, retinoids can actually reduce the amount of pre-cancers in later years for those who have had a more than prudent amount of unprotected sun exposure in their earlier years."

Antioxidants

Antioxidants are what I call the "fertilizer" of the skin. Because your body has limited ability to transfer the benefits of oral antioxidants directly to the skin, topical antioxidants used directly on the skin are a good idea. Once again, a health care practitioner can best guide you to the product (or combination) that will enhance your skin rejuvenation and healing.

There are many options in the world of antioxidants. Two of the most familiar are vitamins C and E, applied directly to your skin.

Unfortunately, as was the case with the glycolics and retinoids, you will not find the really good antioxidants over the counter. A licensed practitioner with expertise in skin rejuvenation will have knowledge of the antioxidants available and can guide you in the selection and combination that will work best for your situation.

Remember, antioxidants alone are not enough. They are best used when in combination with a glycolic or retinoid product.

PART SEVEN

Common Skin Problems and Treatment Procedures

Brown Spots
Red Veins
Wrinkles
Crows Feet
Smoker's Lines
Vertical Line(s)
(Between the Eyebrows)
Forehead Lines
Other Facial Lines
Dull Skin

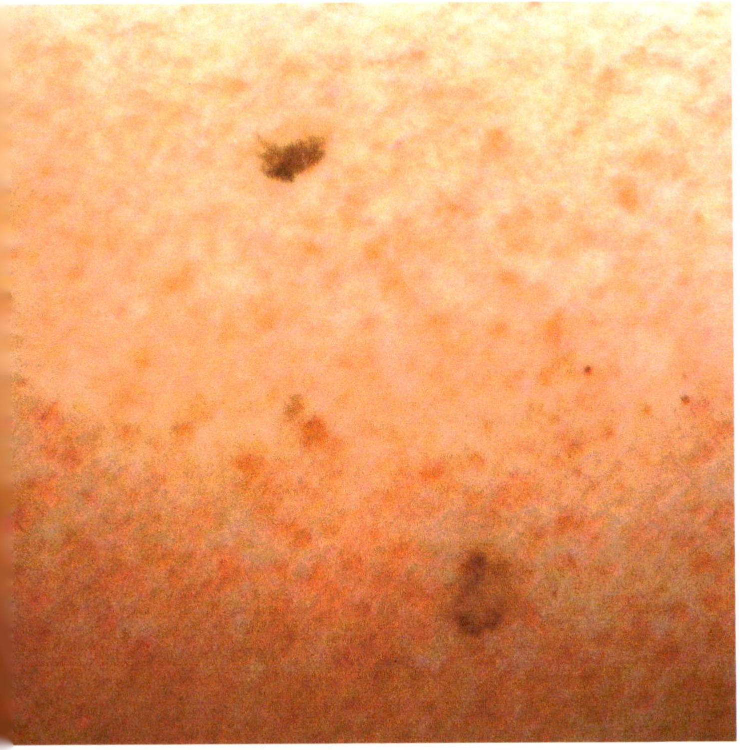

Brown Spots

Brown spots have been called by many names throughout the years—none of them very flattering. They are known as lentigines, age spots, sun spots, liver spots, and a host of other somewhat personalized terms that folks use. They arise from earlier sun exposure and tend to keep coming, even if you're currently avoiding the sun.

On your body, you will notice areas (breasts, buttocks, etc.) that are free of this discoloration. That's because that part of your skin has not been exposed to the harmful UV rays.

These spots may be flat (macular) or elevated (known as seborrheic keratoses, or SK for short). This rather long word is derived from the keratin we talked about earlier. SK's are areas that contain an increased amount of keratin and tend to hyper-pigment (get darker). They even pick up your self-tanner and become even darker. Naturally at this point I hope that self tanner is your sole method of getting a tan.

An SK can be identified in most cases by its dull surface, and an unusual pattern, much like a turtle shell. These lesions are benign (non-cancerous), but are most annoying as they are difficult in some cases to get rid of.

How to Get Rid of Them:

- Photorejuvenation with Intense Pulsed light—commonly referred to as IPL (one may need several treatments of IPL as it's generally not a one-stop solution).
- Alexandrite lasers or lasers targeting pigment.
- Fractionated lasers (you will need several treatments, unless you're using a "big gun" such as a Co2 laser).
- TCA (trichloro acetic acid) peel applied to area.
- Combinations of hydroquinone (bleaching agent) with a retinoid (to allow better penetration).
- Lower-level (non-medical) treatments, such as peels or microdermabrasion treatments. These may take a LONG time.

You and your practitioner will need to work together to ascertain what your needs are and what is the best solution for you.

Before

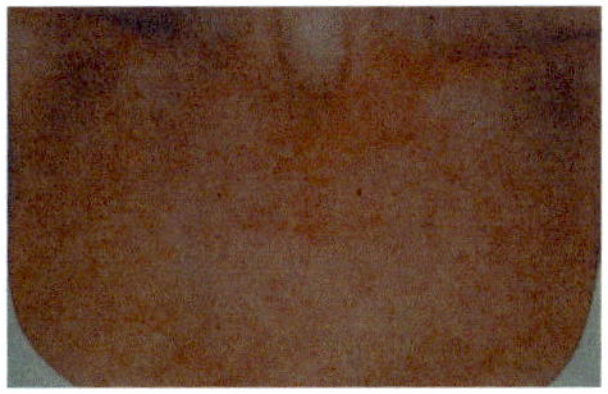

After

Red Veins

Red vessels, otherwise known as telangiectasia, (yeah—say that five times fast) are actually arterioles (tiny arteries) that are dilated (enlarged). This type of problem is hard to permanently erase. Arterioles are under higher pressure with greater resilience than veins. Sun exposure will certainly increase their creation. Steroid use for treatment of such issues as seborrheic dermatitis, etc., can also contribute to their production.

Red vessels on your face or other skin areas may depend upon your genetic makeup (the ancestry issue again!), previous sun exposure, skin disorders, or history of product or medicine usage. For instance, people of Irish/Scottish ancestry, and other northern European descents, are more likely to show tiny red vessels on their face.

The tiny red vessels occur most often around the nose area, but may spread to the cheeks and entire face, depending upon severity. This redness may be triggered by menopause, or emotional flushing. In patients who have been diagnosed with Rosacea, a skin condition said to affect 45 million people worldwide, spicy foods, alcohol, hot beverages, and exercise are frequent triggers of red flushing. No matter the reason for your redness, whether genetics, sun damage, or rosacea, there are methods to work toward alleviating the signs of these unsightly intrusions on your skin.

Treating the overall structure with a light source (not just the reddened spots) will most likely yield a better outcome than trying to hit the tiny vein or spot itself with an injectable. Unfortunately, treatments can eradicate or shrink the offenders, but they often reappear and will need to be re-treated when they return.

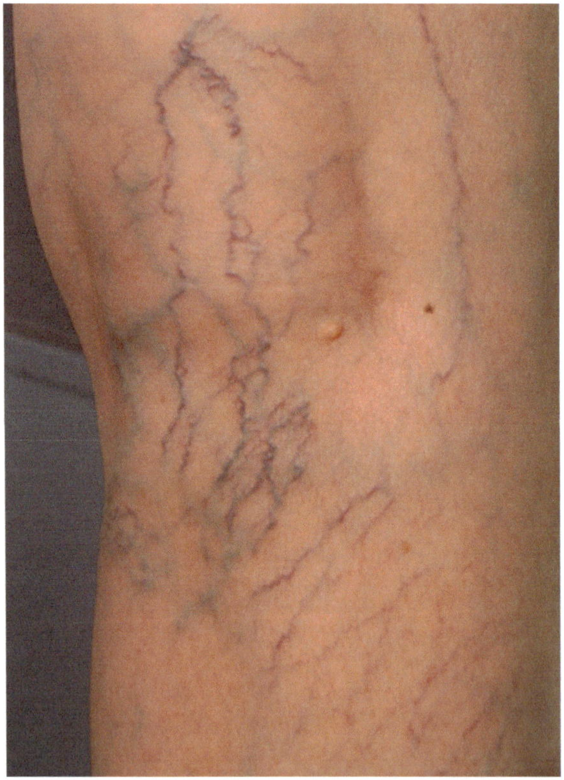

What You Can Do Now

Always, ALWAYS use a sunscreen containing zinc, and perhaps titanium. Contact me for the best currently on the market.

Some topical drugs you can purchase will reduce the redness (they are actually rosacea medications), but they're probably not much help in taking away the actual vessels. But again, they will improve the overall appearance because they lessen the redness. Some drugs I have seen used include:

- Clenia®
- Finacea®
- Metrogel®
- Noritrate®
- Oracea® (this is taken orally)
- Sulfacet-R®

All the above-mentioned medications require a prescription, so you will need to contact your practitioner to obtain them. There are also some topical over-the-counter antioxidant products that may help. Contact me if you wish to learn more.

Another avenue of treatment we spoke about earlier uses lasers and light source procedures. Some of these methods are known by the following trade names or abbreviations:

- Pulse Dye Lasers
- Intense Pulsed Light (to some degree)
- Nd:Yag Lasers (neodymium-doped yttrium aluminum garnet)
- Electrical Desiccation
- RF Ablation (removal of material by radio frequency)

All of these named are standard, evidence-based methods of at least keeping these tiny red veins under control. Arterioles are a continual issue, and one that you may find is with you for life.

"There is no 'remove once and for all' cure. But, if you work with your practitioner, you can keep anyone from knowing you have the problem!"

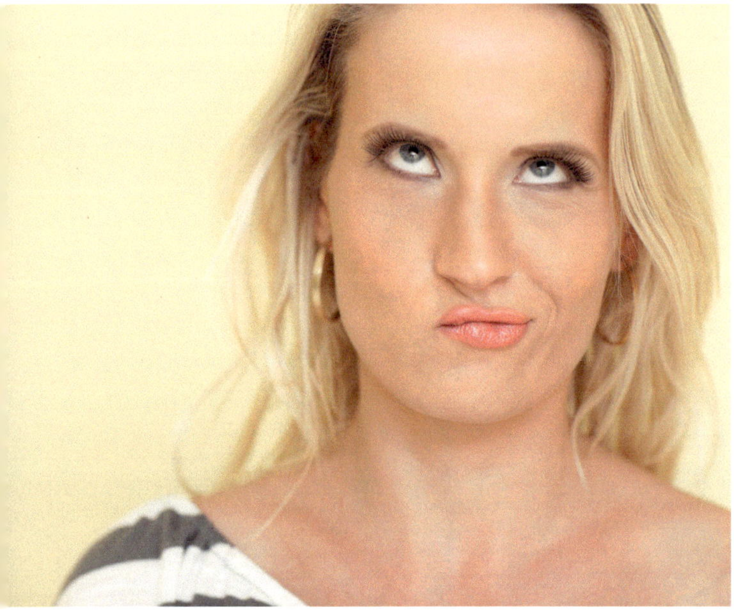

Wrinkles

Wrinkles are actually rhytids. That term may be new to you, but medically that's what your wrinkles are called. The term "rhytidosis" refers to one having many wrinkles of the face disproportionate to their age. What I see in my practice most often is a large amount of wrinkles usually due to excessive sun exposure in earlier years. Heredity also plays a factor. Believe it or not, the way you "make faces" also plays a big part. Some folks use their faces to make all sorts of contortions with their expressions.

Your mom told you your face would freeze that way, didn't she! It is a habit learned over time that can be changed. If you work at a desk all day, put a little mirror in front of yourself and glance as you talk on the phone or type at the computer. My husband discovered the more he worked at his computer, the more his jaw hurt. He found he was clenching his teeth as he concentrated on the monitor, leading to discomfort in his jaw. The same thing happens with facial expressions. You may be unconsciously making an expression, as you frown or squint during the day, causing lines to get a foothold in your facial features.

Crow's Feet (Peri-orbital Rhytids)

We get these lines due to continuous dynamic muscle movement of the obicularis oculi muscle, the muscle partially responsible for moving your lids when you squint, wink, or make many other expressions.

After years of making similar movements, the dermal (collagen) layer of your skin adapts and "settles in" to these patterns. This didn't happen as a child because our dermal layer reproduced faster, and we had much more elastic resistance. In our early 30's this begins to change.

I know, I am just full of good news!

The best treatment for crow's feet is the old standby for facial wrinkles—Botulinum toxin type A. This is the neuromuscular relaxant known mainly by the trade name BOTOX® Cosmetic.

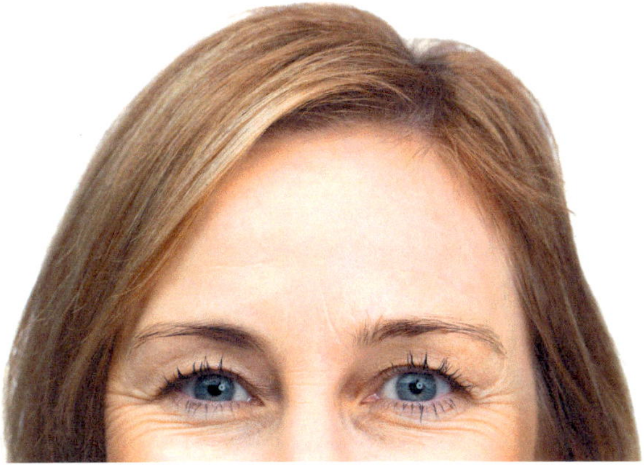

Another great product I've had fabulous results with is known as Dysport®. This neuromuscular relaxant is made by Medicus®. It has been available in Europe and other countries for some time, but has only been used in the U.S. since early 2009.

People often ask me how BOTOX® Cosmetic and Dysport® work. Since these products are neuromuscular relaxants, their sole purpose is to relax the muscle. When the muscle is relaxed (paralyzed essentially), the wrinkle disappears. If your face won't make the crow's feet crunch up and down, then that area will look smooth and wrinkle-free. Keep in mind, you didn't "fix" the problem, you just relaxed the muscle so much it can't make the wrinkle. Once the muscle movement has been relaxed, I use other treatments such as adding a retinoid, which may somewhat extend the life of a neuromuscular relaxant treatment. (Essentially this can save you money by making your BOTOX® Cosmetic injection last longer before you need another treatment.) The typical BOTOX® Cosmetic or Dysport® injection can have results that last anywhere from three to six months, so the longer the better! The retinoid helps your overall appearance by re-growing cells and giving the skin more elasticity as the relaxant keeps the muscle relaxed.

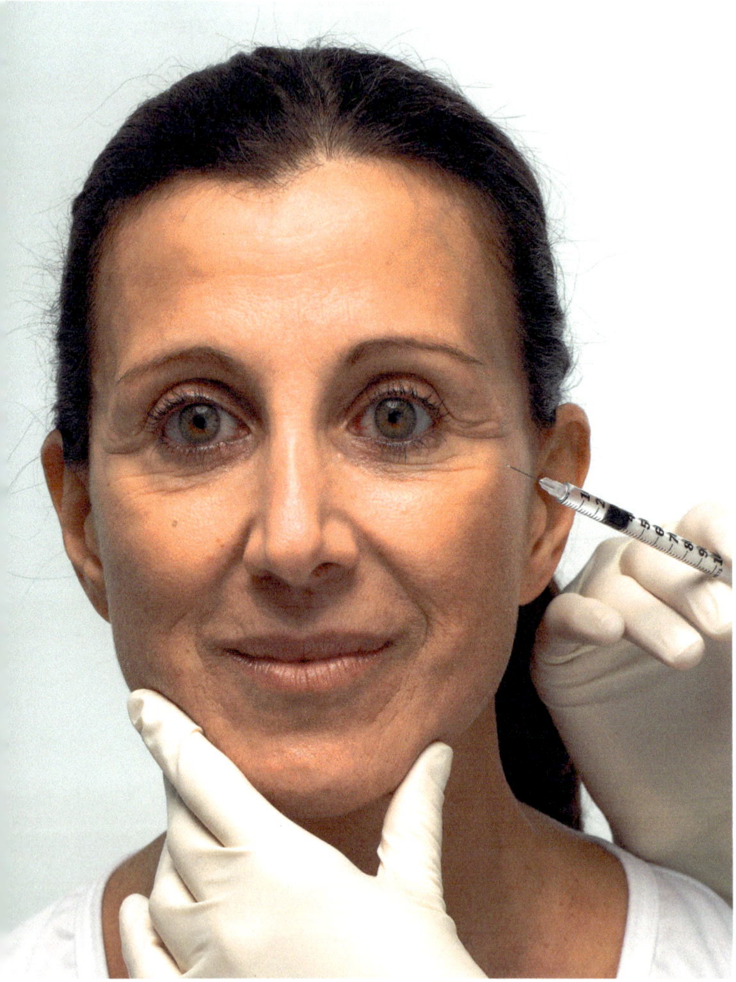

Like all skin care, tiny wrinkles are highly individual. In my own case, I use a tiny bit of BOTOX® Cosmetic for my crows feet, but very seldom. I want small lines when I smile. I personally think it looks less "stiff." When I start to get too many lines, I will simply treat them carefully and should be good to go for a long time.

This brings up a very important point. I am extremely careful in determining what my patients want *before* we begin any treatment. If they want no expression (*which I strongly do not recommend*), then we treat as soon as they begin to see small lines in repose (when their face is in a relaxed, non-expressive state). If they want some expression lines along the side of the eyes when smiling, then we wait longer and/or treat less aggressively. I want my patients to look as natural as possible. Though aging is a part of life, we don't have to look old. But we do want to look human—not like a plastic Barbie doll. Have an idea in your mind of exactly what you expect to see in the mirror after treatments. *Be very clear to your provider what you want, and then, before any procedure is administered, you'll both know you're on the same page to accomplish your goals. Remember—it is your face—not the doctor's.* It is you who has to live with your new look and see yourself in the mirror every day. So I can't state strongly enough how much I urge my patients to be clear in their goals so that I can give them what <u>they</u> want.

Smoker's Lines (Peri-oral Rhytids)

These are the lines around the mouth radiating from the lips outward, like sun rays in a drawing of the sun. You see these lines every day in smokers since they "pucker" as they smoke their cigarettes.

Unfortunately, being a non-smoker doesn't guarantee you won't get these lines. The problem is your mouth. It is a sphincter. Before you say "THAT'S GROSS," here's a definition:

Sphincter: *a circular muscle that normally maintains constriction of a natural body passage or orifice.*

I know it may not be the most pleasant thing you were ever told, but it's true.

This circular muscle acts just like all the other muscles we've discussed. When you're eating, drinking, talking, and even when you're thinking, your mouth forms tiny movements. You may notice people that "pucker" their lips (or mouth) when concentrating. They will eventually get wrinkles around their mouth, just as a smoker will. The easy solution is to stop thinking. Unfortunately, that's pretty hard to do, because we even think and make faces in our sleep. There are, however, things we can do to counteract these irritating (and aging) lines. A simple, but short-lived treatment is a bit of neuromuscular relaxant placed expertly.

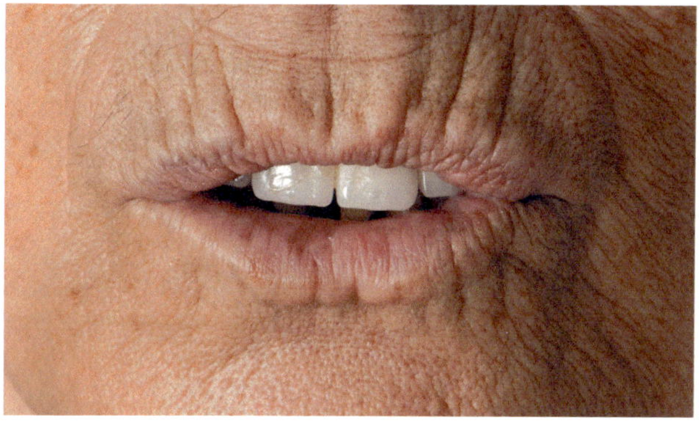

"After years of making similar movements, the dermal (collagen) layer of your skin adapts and 'settles in' to these patterns."

"As a trainer for BOTOX® Cosmetic, I can tell you the mouth area is one of the most challenging injections. What you want to do is 'diminish,' not stop, that movement."

Having done this procedure a multitude of times, I can tell you the lines will decrease or sometimes disappear if they are done correctly, especially ones relatively new. That's the good news.

But if you have significant sun-damage with deep and plentiful lines...a neuromuscular relaxant is not enough. That's when we get out fillers for lines around the mouth. But, again, we need to be careful.

Some providers will fill these wrinkle lines around the lips with a hyaluronic acid (HA) in hopes of pushing the lines out. This sometimes has disastrous results and constitutes a "bad fix." Yes, they may have removed the wrinkles, but

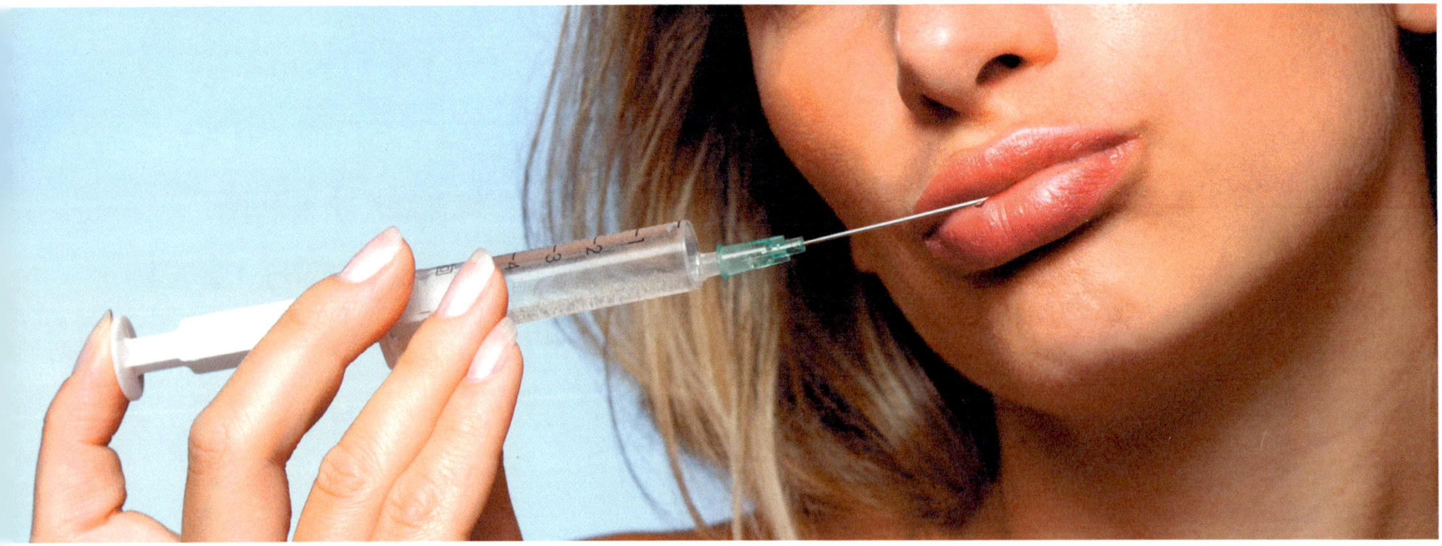

now you are left with severely rounded upper lips (virtually no lip border) and the "platypus" shaped upper lip. The look is not desirable, nor is it one you should expect.

An experienced and skilled practitioner will want a sense of naturalism that brings out your beauty. That's what you're looking for, not someone who will leave you with a fat lip but no wrinkles. You don't want people staring at you asking who gave you a fat lip, do you? They'll be calling the domestic abuse hotline for fear their friend is getting knocked around. And here you've paid good money for that look!

My advice to you—stay away from anyone who can't show you their before and after pictures if they're putting fillers near your lip borders. It takes a very skilled practitioner to do this type of injection, and you should consider only using the best for this procedure!

With that warning, let me now say that fillers do work and I love using them.

The better filler alternatives include Sculptra®, Evolence®, collagen, and other well-known treatments. Some require more expertise than others. Sculptra®, for instance, does require a bit more.

You should ask your practitioner how much of any particular injectable they have done. Then make a wise, informed decision.

Vertical Line (or Lines) Between the Eyebrows

These are sometimes called angry 11's, or angry 1's. On some people, these lines can run very deep and create a most disturbing appearance. They can make you look angry all the time and portray a negative face. The look can suggest worry, frustration, anxiety, or remorse. Some women start to see them early on, and may be as young as 25. If you're one of the luckier ones, you'll not notice these lines until you're well into your 40's. This young lady came in when she noticed the center indentation between her eyebrows getting deeper. After treatment, the indent disappeared.

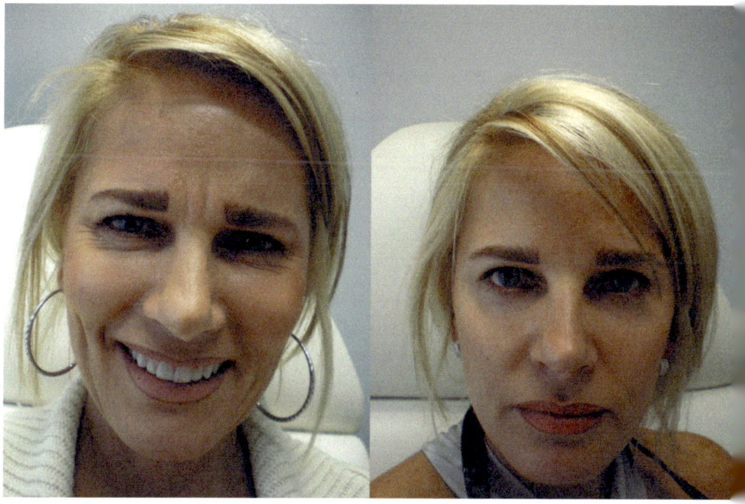

Although she was a beautiful girl when she came in, we were able to stall what was an inevitable effect of facial "maturing."

Men, on average, tend to develop forehead lines first, but lines between the eyebrows definitely leave their mark at some point. In many cases, treatment with a neuromuscular relaxant is enough. In other cases, you may need the area filled with a collagen, HA (hyaluronic acid), or calcium-based product to achieve full correction (meaning total loss of the line). I usually try BOTOX® Cosmetic or Dysport® first, in order to adequately assess the remainder of the crease. The good news is that these lines are quite fixable.

Forehead Lines

These are also related to muscle strength and heredity. Some folks can be in their 40's before they worry about these things. Others see them in their early 20's and find them horrendous. While lines can be filled with light HA's, or the collagen built up with stimulants such as Sculptra®, the best and most immediate answer is a neuromuscular relaxant. In most cases, the lines will smooth out completely.

There is one question almost always asked regarding BOTOX® Cosmetic, Dysport®, or any neuromuscular relaxant: "How will it feel?" I describe the feeling, from personal experience, as having Saran® wrap on my forehead for the first week after it takes effect. After that—it feels totally normal. It is not painful at all, and as the effects are taking place (generally a two-week period elapses before you see the final results) you don't even notice it.

Other Facial Lines

Lines happen on various areas of the face from dynamic muscle movement and lax skin being manipulated by movement. One area specifically prone to indentation (also caused by your inherited facial structure) are the naso-labial folds (the lines going from the sides of your nose to the corners of your mouth. As they begin to indent, they can make you look older than you really are. On the right is a before and after photo of a young lady with this problem.

In addition, both crepe-like skin and "basket-weave" patterns occur most often due to past sun exposure and in areas of extreme thinness. For example, the skin under your eye is extremely thin and this is where you most often see crepe-like wrinkles. If you're a contact wearer, the constant pull on your lower lid can accelerate the problem.

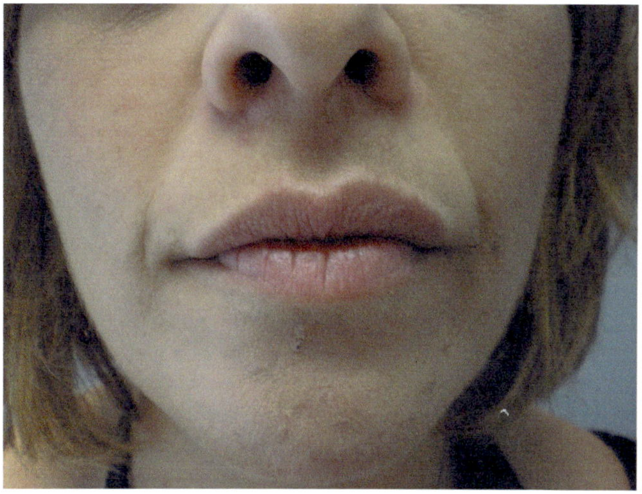

Before

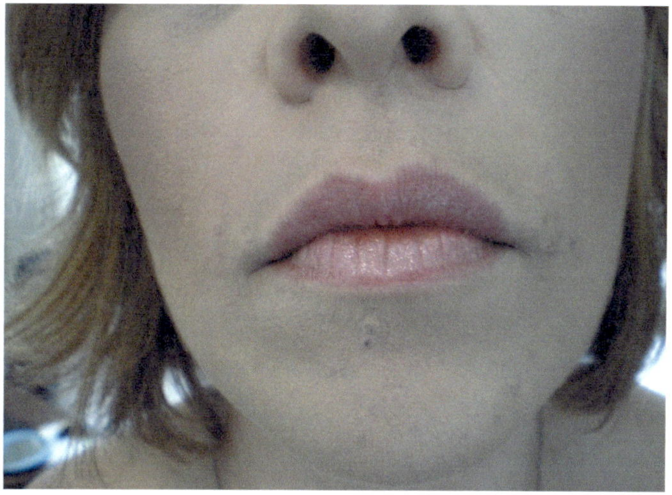

After

Or maybe you're a fan of waterproof mascara, which takes more effort to remove and causes you to wipe harder on your upper and lower eye area. All of these movements and interactions will lead to more wrinkles. But don't despair—you don't have to go buy glasses or give up your long lashes because there is hope. These problem lines can be helped though laser and light devices, evidence-based topical daily skin treatments, or more intense peels that penetrate deep into the dermis. Your practitioner can best decide what will help based on all the factors we discussed earlier, what the office offers, and your desires. But be aware, not all offices offer the latest advances or the best options for a certain condition. You need to research options and get opinions based on consultations with practitioners. And ask your friends who they recommend and why they're happy with their provider. I don't want to minimize the importance of research here. If you were buying a car, you'd look for the best vehicle and the best price—not necessarily the best salesman. But you're not buying a car here—we're talking about your face! So the person who is administering the product and promising you the product needs to be excellent. Many times the best deals aren't the best choice in the long run. You don't want a "lemon," you want top notch quality!

At this time, the products listed below are the most widely used and accepted in addressing wrinkles (now you know they are rhytids). Product choice is usually based on many factors including skin depth and location of the offending area.

- BOTOX® Cosmetic
- JUVÉDERM® Ultra
- Evolence®
- Dysport®
- JUVÉDERM® Ultra Plus
- Artefill®
- Restylane®
- Radiesse®
- Perlane®
- Sculptra®

This list is by no means exhaustive, and the product chosen will depend upon your practitioner's expertise, your individual needs, the site location, and budgetary issues.

"The bottom line? Lines can be greatly remedied, if not totally removed, with proper treatment."

Dull Skin

Dull skin is a bit difficult to quantify and measure. Most folks describe dull skin as skin that "does not glow," "looks pale," "looks lifeless," "is not dewy," and on and on.

The real reason skin looks dull is because it has had too much UV radiation and lacks vascular nutrition underneath. UV radiation destroys all healthy things in skin.

Another reason for dull skin is smoking. UV radiation and smoking have incredible abilities to create harmful free radicals, as we talked about earlier. Therefore, if your goal is to find treatments that will improve your look, and eliminate further free radical damage—it's important to stay out of the sun unprotected, and to quit smoking. When these have been accomplished, you can now focus on regenerating the collagen layer in the dermis. This is the layer that has the actual blood supply. Treatments include collagen stimulants (Sculptra®, Radiesse®), alpha-hydroxy acids, other exfoliation methods (to limited degrees), and antioxidants.

Tried and true mainstay retinoids:

- Retin-A®
- Tretinoin® (generic Retin-A®)
- Retin-A Micro®
- Avage®
- Tazorac®
- Differin®

Those using a retinoid will almost always have significantly better and healthier skin, verified by biopsy or simple examination. One needs to understand, and should look to their provider to furnish proper education regarding how much time may be necessary to adjust to one of these fabulous youth enhancers.

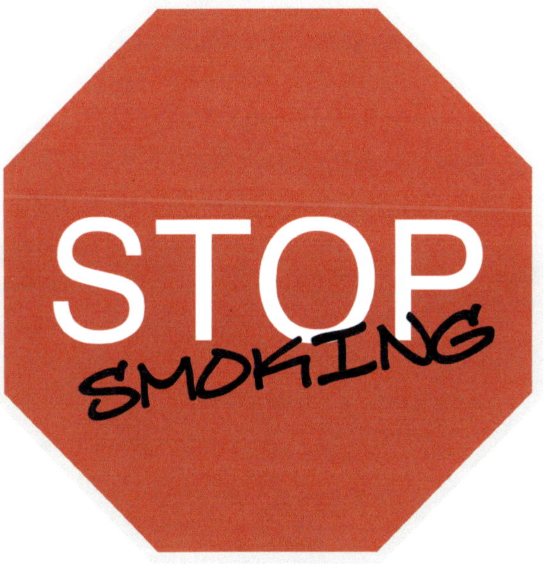

"Once you have experienced the magic of retinoids, you will never look back. This evidence-based treatment is one of the stellar methods to achieve erasing years off your appearance and looking beautiful right now."

PART EIGHT

Let Your Inner Beauty Come Out

The first part of this book examined all the ways we take care of our visible beauty. We've discussed numerous options that can be applied to our skin and overall health regimen. Ultimately, by practicing these things, we can affect our outward appearance.

I've shared with you top secrets on how celebrities manage to always look refreshed and young, while telling you about treatments and procedures that can have you achieving the same results.

And while I love revealing those secrets on how to make you more Beautiful Right Now, I feel it's important to spend some time telling you one more crucial thing. While all that information on skin care and healthy living is valuable—it's not all you need to know to be beautiful.

The phrase "you can't judge a book by its cover" is a very true statement. Because no matter how gorgeous you are on the outside, if you don't feel beautiful on the inside, it is those feelings that will ultimately come through.

We are not simply skin hair and nails—we are so much more! And for you to truly reflect that real beauty, it must come from within.

I know that these can be tough issues, but self-esteem, confidence, and even self-branding (though many don't know exactly what that means...yet) are things I hear about every day in my practice. I witness daily how important these things are in molding our entire persona.

Ask Yourself the Hard Questions

Ask yourself these questions. When you do, don't be flippant. Really think about it and then take a hard look at your answers. You may even want to write your answers. Don't worry, no one can read your mind, or what you have written—so if you find you don't like what you have to say to yourself, then you're already one step closer to self-improvement! Better to be honest than to lie to yourself.

1. Do you like yourself? Be honest. If you don't like yourself, why would anyone else?

2. If you dislike the way you feel inside, why haven't you sought change? If you have, why did you not succeed?

3. Do you blame others for things wrong in your life? Do you blame your parents, your spouse, your kids, or an abuser for decisions that in reality, you've made?

4. If you could change one thing in your life, what would it be? Why?

Okay, now with those answers, let's look at how to make some real positive changes in your life. Whether you want to lose weight, stop smoking, or simply be more patient, tell yourself the time to start is ***now***. Maybe you've determined you should party less, travel more, save more, or take some classes. I don't know what motivates you. But *you* do!

"We are not simply skin hair and nails—we are so much more! And for you to truly reflect that real beauty it must come from within."

"Discover what you love and enjoy, and then ask yourself—"Have I been doing what I love and enjoy?" If not—why not? You alone were given this life and no one else can live it for you. Make it a point to discard all the unhealthy things inside you. Banish the things you hate and gravitate persistently toward a more positive and happy you."

That first step may be the hardest, but it is also the beautiful beginning to your success.

When you self-analyze your feelings, do you find yourself wandering in your past—over and over? Are you saying things that sound like, "But look at what he did to me. I was victimized, I was left. I was abused. I..." (Fill in the blank here with whatever you want). **But this is one story you can, and desperately need to rewrite.** Yes, it happened to you. I so wish I could take it away. Unfortunately, bad things happen to good people. And while we never want it to be us, we must still realize it happens and can be overcome. There are many people who have been able to triumph through it all, and then use those experiences to further improve their life and make it even better—<u>not despite it, but because of it</u>. This is in no way negating your past. So many of my patients have had pasts that are extremely difficult to even listen to, much less live through. The fact that you are here means you are a survivor. You will continue to survive. I want to help you survive more happily.

The popular movie *Soul Surfer* is an example of a hardship unmatched by most of us. A young girl surfing in the ocean had her entire arm bitten off by a shark. She could, as many of us would have, mourned her loss, given up her dreams in despair of her loss, and lived as a *victim* for life.

But instead she persevered, chose positive paths, and now there's a Hollywood movie about her life. She has become a valuable inspiration to millions! What if your story can do something like that? A story meant to be shared. One that could be used to not only improve your life, but help others in the process. Your blessings from this result would be insurmountable!

I'm certainly not claiming to know all the answers. No one does. And I will never make light of anyone's hurts or experiences—**but I encourage you to use your past (we each have our own, some ugly, some not, and most in between) and own it for today.**

By taking ownership (this doesn't necessarily mean we caused it in any way or even participated in it) of all things that have happened in our lives—good and bad—we can use it to better mold our lives and truly make it our own.

So I'll ask another somewhat difficult question: "Do you often find yourself focusing on what you *don't* have?"

Sheryl Crow made a great statement in her song "Soak up the Sun." It stated simply, "It's not having what you want...It's wanting what you've got." This is not in reference to abusive relationships and unacceptable situations. It is in relation to those of us who focus on what we *don't have*. Many times we don't have these things for a reason. Often reasons we cannot foresee, but see later in life. Unfortunately, many believe in the "grass is greener on the other side" concept. I believe that is what these profound lyrics are describing.

I'll dive into this a bit later on. Right now, we are talking about recent or current hurts, injuries, and moving in a positive direction. If you don't do this—if you don't save yourself, you will drown because of another's real or perceived domination over you. This control can be in your body, your mind, or both.

So, let's try ***changing direction.*** We've probably all heard the story of the guy who grimaced as he walked along the gravel road moaning because he felt the stones beneath him. He complained because he had no shoes. He was miserable and bitter, thinking how life had treated him so unfairly. He wondered why he had to go through his day without a pair of shoes. Until he met a man with no feet traveling on that same road, forced to drag his body through the rocks and dirt.

See the change? Many of us can find something, even in the midst of your troubles, to be thankful for. If you have a roof over your head, running water, a means of transportation and food in your fridge, you're wealthier than 90 percent of the world already. And, those 90 percent are not worrying about past relationships, personal hardships, or out-of-touch loved ones.

They are worried about how to put a morsel of something edible in their child's mouth today. This does not mean our issues are not important. They are. It's just that there is a huge correlation here that should not be overlooked. Just being able to not worry about today's meals is a blessing so many do not have. This does not diminish your situation, it's just meant to put it in a perspective of what is really important.

I, like everyone else, feel down and depressed from time to time. That's a normal part of our lives. It can and should be a way to re-evaluate where we go next. But if you stay in that room of despair or sorrow too long, you'll find the door to get out is stuck, and it's hard to get out. Turn on the lights and gaze at the illuminated blessings you have—family, your health, security or all of these. Then break out of that room and scream at the top of your lungs:

"I am more than my past. I am more than my experiences. I am a person in charge of my life!"

That release is the biggest beauty lift you can give yourself—and it doesn't cost a dime or come in a syringe or fancy bottle.

Open The Package

To truly have your inner beauty shine through, you need to open that outer package and shine. If you were a present, how would others see you? What is your wrapping like?

I've got a friend who is, figuratively speaking, wrapped in the brightest, shiniest, metallic wrapping paper she could find. Bows, glitter and ribbons are what I see when I picture her. And she's so much fun. I want to open her up and find out what's on the inside because it simply is too inviting to ignore it. You want to discover all that is beneath the decorative wrap. You're intrigued with her outer shell and you want more.

But then I have another friend. Her wrapping paper is more like a faded, simple tan shipping paper. There are no ribbons or bows. And even the tape holding down the seams looks ratty and dirty.

Both are great women and I love them both dearly, but one is extremely outgoing, friendly, full of life, and eager to experience the world and enjoy living. The other is extremely shy. She never wants to draw attention to herself because her self-esteem is so low. She's afraid of interaction with others and is always looking at the negative side of things out of fear. Though I do spend time around her—it must be for short periods of time—because her chronic negativity will wear anyone down. She is nice, open, and I love her, but after the experience, you feel like the life has just been ruthlessly sucked out of you. She exudes need.

I can spend fun weekends with my shiny, wrapped friend and wonder where the time went, but my plain-Jane friend has me looking for an escape route after only twenty minutes in her company. Not because I don't treasure her, but because I am exhausted.

So what is the difference between these two ladies? You can't blame it on their appearance; both are naturally attractive, smart, and healthy women. And to further complicate the matter, both were abused as children. But one decided to take charge of her life, get some help about what happened, and not live victimized by the past. She chose to relish each day with happiness and new expectation. The other lives completely in the past. She blames her current situation and choices on things that happened years ago and were totally out of her control. She spends several hours of most days reliving events she found extremely hurtful. She is not alone...many people do this. Reliving events, even if they occurred thirty years ago, keeps them in the *present.* That keeps them happening day after day, hour after hour. It prevents anyone who is engaging in this behavior from moving on to a happy, safe life. **She needs to take back her life and finally experience the present.**

There is only one thing that we, as human beings in our lives on this earth, have control over: <u>Our Thoughts</u>. This puts us far ahead of any other species. We are designed that way so we can protect ourselves from bad things, and elevate ourselves when we realize we can do better. If we wish to go downhill, we can guide our thoughts to the negative and go there. If we wish to do better, our success, triumph, and resulting euphoria begins with a single, positive thought. It's that simple.

Do You Like Yourself?

I often compliment my friends, and yet many times I find that as soon as they hear something positive about themselves, they immediately respond with a negative. This shows they may have some self-esteem issues. When someone says you are pretty, do you say, "Thank you?" Do you then smile and feel good about it? Or do you look down, and say, "No, I really don't"...and then go on and on with a litany of reasons why you don't deserve the compliment. Or more accurately, cannot *accept* the compliment.

If you are guilty of this, examine it now. Try to appreciate the sincerity of the sender, respect it for its sincerity, and finally relish in it, even if only for a minute. Unless you have something terribly attractive (you know, money, a good job offer, a gift of some sort to give) that you feel they are fishing for, then accept it as a sincere comment. Live in the moment. But if you don't do this, examine why. Appreciate how you look to others and that someone notices you. Learn to feel you actually ***deserve*** the compliment. You have to get to know and love yourself before others can reciprocate.

If you ever find yourself wishing you had been nicer or maybe less snappish with someone, ask yourself how that probably made you appear to them. More importantly, how did that make *them* feel? Let's remember that *everyone* is in a state of dealing with something. Hurting someone else will eventually hurt us more. Were you trying to appear confident, but not bossy? Were you trying to appear in control and in charge and that's why you spoke or reacted the way you did? Well, maybe while you were trying to appear confident, do you think you really just came off as arrogant? This is not the exuding of confidence. It is the constant drip of a low self-esteem. Confidence says to the world you are comfortable in your own skin... but it never degrades others in the process.

Here's an example: I've got an acquaintance who is young, fit, beautiful, and has a law degree. She is the envy of every woman's eye when she walks into a room. *Until she opens her mouth.* And no, I don't mean she has horrible teeth, bad breath or an atrocious accent. It's how she comes across. *She acts like a complete expert on everything.* You simply can't get two words in, and if you are lucky enough to do it, take care to not contradict her, or you'll pay by her badgering you into submissiveness until you agree or retreat. I watched one man after another strike up a conversation with her, and then suddenly check their phone, glance at their watch, remember an important email they need to make, and then escape. They were not only turned off by her aggressiveness, they were probably willing to hang themselves to get out of the situation. She can be even worse with women whom she sees as competition.

"What does this mean in a nutshell?

Just Be Real—to yourself and to others."

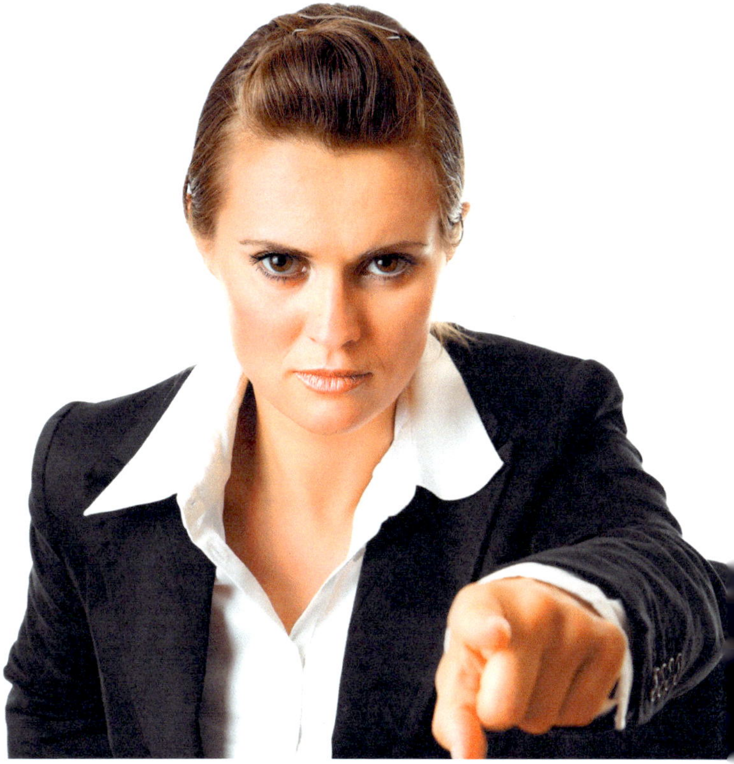

And be kind if your opinions differ from someone else's. One of my favorite lines is, "Let's just agree to disagree." I think the world would be a more pleasant place if more people followed that motto. Let's face it: you're never going to please everybody. But if you start with yourself and accept yourself and don't hide behind insecurities, excuses, or false airs, people can see the real you underneath. That's where real beauty can shine through.

PART NINE

Celebrity Envy

People often aspire to be famous. Some desire the recognition, others the lifestyle they lead, and many simply want the money. Of course—most people I talk to want all three! But I caution you in thinking they have it all! I have many celebrity friends and believe me, it's not all a box of chocolates, as Forrest Gump would say.

One thing most of my more-famous friends miss is their privacy. Can you imagine what it must be like to be continually stalked by the paparazzi? Envision trying to go out for a quiet dinner without having to be interrupted several times to sign autographs. Or say you want to take your toddler to the park and swing them without being harassed?

Imagine your life being the focus of every *Entertainment Tonight* show or celebrity magazine subscription. Oh, it may sound great in the beginning. You picture yourself wearing a beautiful ball gown from Versace, dripping in diamonds and walking the red carpet to accept your award…

but think about the other hundreds of non-red carpet days in a year.

When I want to exercise, I throw my hair in a ponytail, apply sunscreen without makeup and heaven forbid—I may even lace up my sneakers without shaving my legs first. Unfortunately for Goldie Hawn, she did the same thing and someone snapped her picture which can now be found on the Internet. Search if you dare.

Believe it or not, there is a certain freedom to anonymity. I can choose to be myself and go for a run whenever I want, wherever I want, and for as long as I want—**in peace.**

Do you think Angelina Jolie, Jennifer Anniston or Princess Kate Middleton can do that?

Of course not—someone is hiding behind the bushes trying to get paid top dollar for the worst photograph they can find in the most unflattering light. And smear campaigns and untruths are perpetrated against these individuals all the time just to sell a few million more copies. The thick skin these celebrities must develop to shield the harmful things the media thrusts at them is almost unimaginable.

Seriously, I don't know how some of my friends keep their sanity day in and day out when the front covers of *US Magazine* have them in a bikini with cellulite blown up to look like a cottage cheese factory, or breasts sagging to their knees as they bend over to pick up their kids'

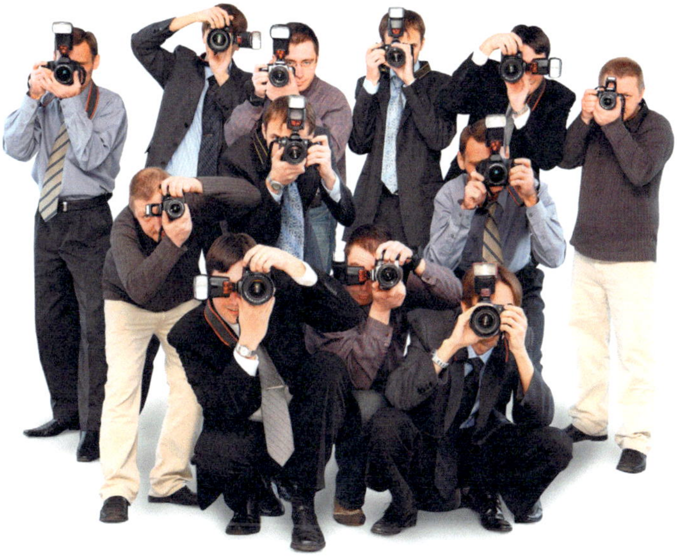

toys. They really don't look that bad in real life. Just as Photoshop can be used to airbrush and make flawless a cover girl, it can also be used to highlight any undesirable quality imaginable. The imagination is the limit.

For the most part, these are people just like you and me, who just happen to have chosen a career very much in the public eye in the entertainment/fashion industry. They don't deserve most of the bad rap they get and they struggle with insecurities and attacks on their looks and character way more than the average person. In a way that's good news to you and me. Because if they can succeed in the distorted magnified view of the paparazzi and the world, then we should be able to feel confident and secure with a lot less scrutiny. Make sense?

So when I give you advice on how to feel confident and feel good in your own skin—bikini or not—know that at least people aren't out there with high-powered cameras ready to catch your bumpy thighs or puffy eyes.

"If you enjoy these celebrity magazines, great—but don't believe everything you see or read, as most of it is manufactured."

Easy Tips You Can Do Right Now

- Just enjoy the life you live. No one can live it for you.
- Feel confident in your own skin. Seek to be beautiful from the inside out. It will show. It will make a difference.
- Improve your demeanor.
- Pay attention to how you carry yourself; notice your gait as you walk. Is it slow or purposeful?
- Hold your head up.
- Stand and walk with your back straight and your chest slightly out. Lead from your hips. Instantly you feel more power with this stance.
- Make eye contact and listen when people talk to you.

Simple Signs to Avoid

- Bad posture.
- Don't interrupt when others are talking. Treat them as if they are the only ones in the room and soon you'll be the finest conversationalist around—without saying a word.
- Don't try to put your experiences in when they're talking about their problems. Don't distract them to tell them what you've been through—this is all about them, not you.
- Know your limits—this is in food, alcohol and love. Do not take abuse from anyone. You deserve respect.
- And lastly, but most important—count your blessings every day.

"Thank you for letting me share. I pray you all find the best in yourself, in your dreams and in all your relationships. I truly believe you can be Beautiful Right Now, inside and out!"

Sincerely,
Bonnie Marting

A CLOSING WORD

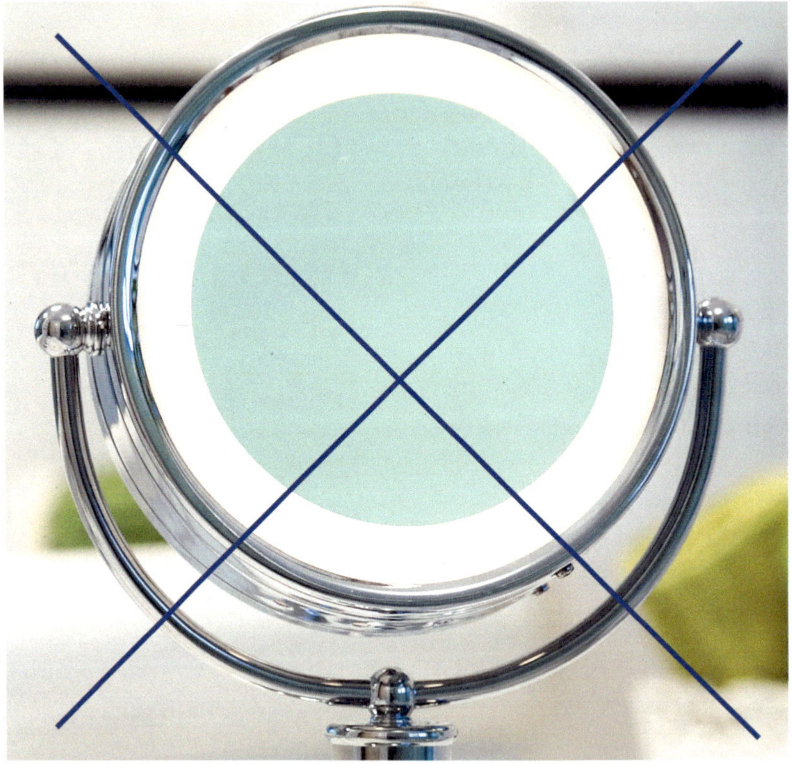

The Dreaded Makeup Mirror

While any skin imperfection can be a concern, please don't sabotage your beauty by going "over the top" with a magnifying mirror. Especially one sold with a built-in light so your skin can look even more flawed!

These horrible magnifiers are like looking under a microscope—making things look two to ten times bigger than they really are. These mirrors not only cause self-deprecation, but can reveal things on your skin that won't be evident in the regular world for years to come, if ever.

Sometimes a patient will point to a spot that I cannot see, no matter how bright the light I am using is. When I ask if they have a magnifying make up mirror, 99.9 percent of the time they say "Yes."

The problem is the magnifying mirror, not the skin. I beg them to go home and throw the thing out.

These magnifying mirrors are great for being able to see well when applying makeup, but please don't frustrate yourself by trying to find imperfections. It will ruin every day before it ever begins. Remember, others see you in real life, not magnified.

Thank you for taking the time to read this book, the first in the BeautifulRightNow.com series. It is my hope that you have been educated and maybe even amused at some of the things we have talked about.

I love what I do, and have been blessed to form many wonderful friendships with my patients. This allows us to talk openly and honestly. A wonderful part of this friendship is watching someone grow more beautiful and confident as we make subtle yet stunning changes that actually change their lives for the better. If there is any way I can help you, please do not hesitate to call on me.

I hope to hear from you soon,
Bonnie

Made in the USA
Monee, IL
05 November 2026

67385915R00038